BIODYNAMICS OF OSTEOPATHY

Phase Seven

Second Edition

James Jealous D.O.

For more information about Dr. Jealous please visit:
https://BiodynamicsOfOsteopathy.com

BIODYNAMICS OF OSTEOPATHY Phase Seven

Hardback ISBN: 979-8-2955-3930-5

Second Edition 2025

James Jealous D.O. (1943–2021) practiced as an osteopathic physician, teacher and writer for many years. His life's work was to found and develop the specific methodology of Biodynamics of Osteopathy, following the lineage of Dr. A.T. Still and Dr. W.G. Sutherland.

This is one of a series of Biodynamics of Osteopathy books. They grew organically from sets of handouts written by Dr. Jealous and given to students during courses taught by him and his teachers. After many years he collected the handouts together and created individual course manuals, which he added to and rewrote many times. After several more years they evolved further into books.

TABLE OF CONTENTS

OSTEOPATHY IS SERVICE

We use our hands ...

To treat the Whole patient

To listen to the indwelling movements of Life

To treat all levels of illness

To assist in building the patient's functional reserve

To support homeostasis and trophicity by balancing the activity of the autonomic nervous system

To explore "laws not framed by human hands" (Dr. Still and Dr. Sutherland)

To cooperate and communicate with the Laws of Nature (Dr. Wales)

"To find the Health" (Dr. Still)

To get to the treatment plan

To get to the diagnosis

To help establish a point of Rest or Neutral around which the Whole can come to balance

To find Cause

We believe ...

We have an innate capacity to heal
The patient functions as a whole
The autonomic nervous system plays a major role in disease and healing
Structure and function are one form of activity
The Divine is indwelling
Life moves beyond death
There is a Constant Movement toward Normal
We are here to Serve Humanity

Normal is ...

"A sense of peace and harmony" (Dr. Sutherland)
Ease of motion, without tension
A capacity for Neutral
A sense of Wholeness to Life
The capacity for adaptation, change without compensation.

"Skill is proportionate to one's understanding of normal" (Dr. Still)

Phase Seven Is Dedicated to the Beloved Robert Fulford, D.O.

He was a teacher who was not afraid to speak openly about Love. He loved children and restricted his practice to helping them.

When I first met him, I asked, "Is the mechanism God?" He answered, in his mystical way, "Turn it around."

He was a student of the Ouspensky school of esoteric Christianity and explored the vibrational theory his whole life.

His gaze was deep and steady.

His heart was open to all.

His hands were like those of a surgeon.

His life was a gemstone for Osteopathy.

Love does not die. Thank you, Dr. Fulford.

THE HEALTH

Phase Seven Highlights the Health

This curriculum, like all the other Phases, has a history behind its content. The light behind this course shines back to Dr. Still and Dr. Sutherland.

Dr. Still's writings are full of adoration for the "perfect," often referring to nature and a supreme intelligence as absolute wisdom.

Dr. Still's very famous comment "Find the Health; anyone can find disease," has plagued many a mind over the last century. As early as 1966, this quote entered my Osteopathic notes ... it has lived and grown within me. Now it resides as the most important task in my life.

The words are clear, but where and what is this Health?

In the first edition of Magoun's *Osteopathy in the Cranial Field*, Dr. Sutherland paraphrases Dr. Still as he draws a picture of the perfect system unimpeded by distortions. This is followed by Dr. Sutherland's own impressions. One needs to review this often (page 15, first edition) and reflect on whether it is poetry, philosophy, or a report of their experiences from many years of watching the movements of life.

Dr. Sutherland's commentaries clearly show how he saw something perfect, unerring, and capable of miraculous (uncanny) transmutations.

He observed liquid light and transparency. He witnessed something breathing through us that cannot be "diminished," something omnipresent. He sees the Breath of Life (April 12, 1948,

Contributions of Thought), a term that echoes throughout the spiritual history of the human race as the movement of incarnating Divine Love. His intimacy was such that he called his creator "Dad."

As the Biodynamic model came into being, there was severe resistance to any comments about the Health. People got very angry ... surprisingly so. The idea was threatening. Why? I do not know, unless somehow it was meaningless for some people ... today there are thousands of Osteopaths who accept the challenge of coming to understand and depend upon Dr. Still's words ... "find the Health."

Still must have found this Health or he would not have made such a demanding comment ... he leaves us no place to go. He says anyone can find disease and insists that the hallmark of our skill is to find something more essential—finding disease is not our professional goal. These are firm words! Still follows this line of commentary when he also tells us many times that our skill depends on our understanding of normal ... this implies that a knowledge of lesions and disease is only where one begins the journey to understand how to think, feel, and know these truths at the core of Osteopathic Principles.

Our profession is not a clone of western allopathic thinking. It is unique in its orientation and principles, all of which reflect the existence of an intelligence beyond our control and beyond the processes of disease. Life depends on Life, on the incarnate motion of the eternal, the infinite.

When we meet this Health, we are changed by its presence. It heals us and awakens our memory.

I always believed in Dr. Still's direction, but the demand it placed on me was persistently making me uneasy and tired ... I felt that I would never see what he was calling us to experience. Even Dr. Sutherland's first words in the first edition of *Osteopathy in the Cranial Field* were a warning from Alexander Pope's poem *An Essay on Criticism*: "A little learning is a dangerous thing; Drink deep, or taste not the Pierian spring." Here again we meet the demanding tones of a mentor. How many of us truly see the point? How many of us will ever come to be Osteopaths of this fragrance?

The depth increases as one journeys along. If we carry the load alone, we will fall ... our consciousness and intention must be given to us by the Health, not from our own self- will ... this reality takes time and the help of good mentors. We do not come into it easily, nor can we conceive of it being clinically more dynamic than techniques framed by human theories.

As I traveled, I met a few teachers who followed the quest to experience what Drs. Still and Sutherland were pointing toward.

Dr. George Laughlin, A. T. Still's grandson, shone his grandfather's light in his words, his deeds, and his teaching. From 1966 to 1970, as I watched him, he demonstrated his understanding. The clinical results he obtained astounded me, as an extern in his office. He was devoted to Still and Sutherland. In 1954, after Sutherland's death, he saved the cranial work almost single-handedly. As the story was told to me by Dr. Day in 1976, the American Osteopathic Association (AOA) notified the schools in the states that if they taught cranial work they would be closed down (something the AOA could do at the time). The cranial people were frightened by the consequences and retreated, but George stepped forward, told the American Osteopathic Association that Kirksville was going to teach a course, and that "they could come and close the Kirksville school down" ... So George scheduled a course ... but no one would help him ... there was fear of personal loss ... however, four persons from the East Coast came to Kirksville to teach and support this work as its life was threatened: Ruby Day, Anne Wales, Chester Handy (Anne's husband), and a Dr. Quint. George Laughlin paid the tuition for eleven students to attend. He also paid for all the teachers' expenses. The course was two weeks long.

The American Osteopathic Association never bothered the cranial work again.

All these teachers demonstrated their conviction, even in the face of losing their livelihoods. I tell this story because they all believed in the depths of Osteopathy. They all clearly knew and trusted the Health without social or political compromise. George, Anne, Chester, and Ruby were all exceptional in their skill. These were persons who had the courage to stand up and face the threat. They were the ones who took something different from Sutherland and continued to discover and dig on for more Health in themselves.

This is a true story. Without these four "warriors" we would have no cranial work to study. It is solely because of their character that we have this teaching ... may they hear our hearts beating with them.

The awareness of the Health was part of an oral teaching rarely placed in print. Many people formed around Dr. Sutherland. They took his courses, taught with him, and created an intimate community around him. Some of these people were Rollin and Alan Becker, Tom Schooley, Drs. Barnes and Hull, Alvera Miller, Charlotte Weaver, Dr. Biddle, Ruby Day, George Laughlin, Chester Handy, Dr. Quint, Robert Fulford, Anne Wales, and some who remain hidden ... they found the treasure buried in the Health and it proved Itself meaningful.

Sometimes the term "the mechanism" was used to describe the supreme intelligence and love found in this ocean of Health. Later, like many aspects of Sutherland's work, the word became cheapened and popularized. Unfortunately, the words became more important than the experience of the indwelling Health. This is true today, as many talk about ideas without direct communication with the reality. One must walk the road a long time before the words become a living presence. Today "everyone knows everything" ... words are toys, power tools, empty. We need to regain integrity in our speech.

Our predecessors were not musculoskeletal specialists but general practitioners ... complete physicians ... Osteopaths. They are the reason these words have true meaning ... we are part of a tradition; much was held for us to inherit, but only if we are sincere about being real

Osteopaths … For many, Osteopathy has died. The teaching about the Health that we inherit is a real challenge, and the means for entering that challenge is the purpose of Phase Seven.

The Health is our conceptual vehicle. It is our beginning, our origin, our original nature. It contains our name and its meaning. It mirrors only who we are; all else we imagine of ourselves is a misunderstanding, a subconscious tension. This tension is the energy of one's image of oneself, and often our identity around this causes despair. One can feel betrayed when the betrayal is in oneself. We fail to see the Health, and this disassociation from the Health is a betrayal of Love.

This false identity can only be appreciated fully when we have been helped by the Health, through its love, to see our state. *The healing does not come from a personal insight of one's self-image but from the Health unveiling one's own true self.*

It is then that one is re-centered in a place of ease. This new sensation of ease with oneself penetrates the physical body, which begins to sense its own nature differently. It feels suspended in life. The brain actually agrees with this new truth and sees the true soma in the Health. Now the sensation of normal shifts toward the true soma. Our sense of soma, as transparent to the Breath of Life, awakens a memory of innocence. This newness is the soul re-identifying its orientation from "self-image" to original image.

This beginning of wholeness can be intense and requires a period of rest and adaptation. The fire of love that burns away the dross is almost too much for the "little mind" to absorb. Time is required before transmutation finishes and one can return to the Health as a friend rather than a personal spiritual goal. One no longer needs to center oneself; the friendship becomes meaningful for its own sake. One feels the sweet love of the presence that has brought one home. One sits by the fire, content to be there with the master of the house. One's sense of time shifts to eternity. The sense of soma is infinitely felt as undying in its nature. Often, food preferences simplify, mirroring an interior renovation of the house that begins with the removal (transmutation) of the contents as they were. The house is emptied of its past content and refurnished with new meaning. Ownership is dismissed. It is the master's house. It is a place of love.

IMAGES OF THE HEALTH

This commentary is about what one sees of the Health after the mind is centered by love.

At eighty-six years of age, Dr. Still said, "I love my patients. I see God in their faces and their form."

To witness the Health in another person, one's senses must be under the influence of the indwelling Health in everything. Neutrality is necessary.

As we are, our senses are usually attached to the will of our ego. We naturally see other persons as projections of our personal formulation, not as living landscapes of Divine beauty. It would not be human to do otherwise.

As we let the Tide center us, a reversal or conversion of the senses eventually occurs, usually over a number of years.

Much of this depends upon our response to the Health when it surfaces in ourselves. If we only see it as an experience and move on, then it will never become a relationship.

The desire of the heart to be with this Majesty must be strong. This does not mean we try hard to be with it, but we accept the companionship of the Health in every moment even if we cannot feel it ... we know it is there.

We make the relationship with the Health flourish by being neutral to our humanity as well as that of others.

To see the Health in another person, the overlay of tensions unrelated to the Divine image must become transparent. One does not look deeper. One knows neutral, and seeing is a consequence.

Transparency of everything to the motion of creation is the idea that can take us to the experience. Imagine that everything is transparent to the Tide of creation ... as it is ... work with this and see what transpires.

The art of seeing the Health is not from personal effort, but rather from the action of the dynamic stillness upon our awareness, after the mind is neutral, desiring nothing. Neutral allows one to be shifted by the Divine, or Deity, as Dr. Becker noted (1965 Sutherland Memorial Lecture).

When the tension of being active or passive is gone, the tensions abate. They are transmuted, and then one feels the blessing of the Divine presence that was already shining.

The principles are simple; the cost is your time to be watchful and neutral.

Dr. Still refers often to mind, motion, and matter. Mind is the mind of the Divine mystery, the mind of creation that animates life and gives it motion.

Matter is the clay of life that the Divine breathes the Breath of Life into. The clay is the substance of the Dynamic Stillness, not the clay one sees on a riverbank. This clay is substantial.

Mind, motion, and matter incarnating as one. The mystery that animates all life unfolds into the diversity of all living things. Holy animation is not man-made, "not framed by human hands." It flows eternally. It is beyond the veil of our self-centered senses. These facts coming from Dr. Still are about what he saw as the Health. Dr. Becker talked about the "veil," about going behind the veil.

Understanding this language helps us think more clearly and not compare one reality with another as if they lay in parallel equalities. Our world is under the veil. We are in lesion, full of tension and asleep to Dr. Still's story.

The world of the Health has no perceptual tension, none.

The direction of ease is the true nature of Life.

Ease is called the "river of life."

Ease opens a space. If we step into that space, we find a welcoming love.

We will see our humanity and others' humanity as superficial to any meaning.

We are not forced by Divine love to obey. It is love that moves us, if we wish.

In the embryo there is no resistance to the blueprint that unfolds.

This is what the Health means in the context of embryology as we have come to know it by listening to the fluid body.

Mind ... matter ... motion ... life unimpeded ... Health

In the first edition of *Osteopathy in the Cranial Field*, Dr. Sutherland collects his views and Dr. Still's into a picture that is clearly composed beyond the veil of the ordinary senses. Their descriptions are from direct knowing, not from ideologies.

Here is what is said ...

Dr. Still: "Motion must be guided and directed by a supreme being, down to the individual cell, or there would be chaos and death."

Then Sutherland continues ...

"Dr. Still understood the cerebrospinal fluid as the highest known element in the human body; he envisioned this fluid as an intermediary in the movement of divine intelligence ... a channeling of creation into embryological segments and irrigating them with life ... giving form and function, order and intelligence to our existence. Without this, there would be only decay and chaos. All life is manifest in this motion" (page 15, paragraphs 1 and 2, first edition of *Osteopathy in the Cranial Field*).

When you have time ... try to feel your way through the above words; each word is a reality.

Still and Sutherland connected the Divine, Osteopathy, Primary Respiration, embryology, and inner harmony into one event ... please notice that this wholeness is transparent ... there is no reference to structure or systems ... this is how the Health feels ... no anatomy. The science of embryology at its best is well behind what these men saw …

On pages 15 and 16 of the first edition of *Osteopathy in the Cranial Field* and again in the April 12, 1948, section of *Contributions of Thought*, Dr. Sutherland brings out another image of the Health.

He describes feeling the cerebrospinal fluid and the Breath of Life (the movement of supreme intelligence).

He feels a spark (fire) that is unerring, intelligent, in command, and superseding all other functions. He therefore called it Primary Respiration and the spark of life.

Again, we have an image without anatomy or systems—wholeness that is moving perfectly (the Health).

This was only seen by Sutherland after he removed force from his observations. He instructs us to get away from palpation and away from our physical senses.

He sees the interchange between creation and the created "Heaven and Earth."

Later in his life, Sutherland asked his wife to paint a picture of his model … it was, as many know, a "House Under the Sea."

It is a picture of the Health … the house is our existence … the body, soul, and spirit living as a house … they are the house, one domain.

The doors and windows are open … no tensions … neutral.

The Tide (in this case, the Breath of Life) moves through the house that it creates and sustains. The house is transparent to the movement of Creation (Love).

In the house is the teacher, the beloved master, the fire of love personified … as we mature in neutral we meet the teacher, and the teacher becomes an intimate friend.

The house has many rooms.

One room is not in the house … it is a false home … inside this false domain, we enter a "void" … a dark room where there is nothing … only our isolation from God, our fears, and our ego … as we come into it … we find only our selfish feelings and emotions … we are alone with our own decay and chaos … the mystics call this place "the dreads" … it is something we all encounter on the way home … as we sit and try to be still, we first encounter our humanity and its unlivable breath … it is dead to life … as we adjust and become neutral to this facet of our humanity, we slowly pass into the first room of the true house.

This void is a hard place. If you are not careful, you can believe that you are a "bad person," especially if your idea of yourself is prideful or vain … this is no-man's-land, a desert that we can cross … the battleground for liberation … finally, we discover a dependency on being centered by the Tide … and struggle to integrate this truth into our work.

Then we come into the house … the meeting place … it is very different from the "void" … one feels like one is in a single room in a house with many rooms … after a while, we begin to understand we are a welcomed guest and that the host is home but resting … we can hear his breathing … this is the other breath we find after breathlessness occurs in some of our meditations. This phase lasts as long as necessary. This meeting or waiting room is peaceful, dark, and restful … one comes to a sense of weariness and rests.

There are other rooms …

THE TEACHING ABOUT THE HEALTH IN BIODYNAMICS

The teaching of Biodynamics is an attempt to bring an inquiry into Osteopathic Principles to a place where the clinician can be taught by the Health.

We begin this journey in Phase One with the recognition of motion present in the lesion field. The basis of the Osteopathic lesion is its motion. The lesion is named by its motion, not by its motionlessness.

As we look for involuntary motion in a lesion field, we find that in spite of the severity of the confinement of the illness there is still something Healthy inside the more obvious "withering field."

This Health in the lesion field is called motion present. Inside the decay and chaos is the "still small voice" of the Health itself.

Our first principle of treatment, therefore, is to "synchronize with the Health (motion present) in the lesion." This initiates a therapeutic process that is controlled by Primary Respiration, not the operator's force.

By the time we come to Phase Two, we have worked with motion present in the lesion enough so that the end point is a neutral in the whole patient. These end points now become the point where treatments begin, not end. This is a dramatic shift in our principles of treatment. In Phase Two we also begin to see the Fluid Body as a unique activity.

As we learn to cooperate with the Fluid Body, we realize that one of its qualities is a stillness. This stillness (level two) is different from the neutral in the whole patient (level one). This stillness activates automatic shifting, an unerring diagnostic/therapeutic continuum, the intelligence of which is an aspect of the Health. The Health has been in touch with the lesion field since its beginning and has prioritized the healing process ... why did it not intervene early?

It needed a neutral (i.e., permission).

Our next step is to learn to trust the Health and its wisdom.

The therapeutic forces generated by the Health have a variety of spatial and temporal dynamics. In Phase Three we meet the Long-Tide and the sea around us. We begin to realize that Zone B is connected to the ocean (Zone D) ... this is why we chose the word "Biodynamic" for our work ... because to both Sutherland and Blechschmidt there is something outside and extragenetic that is controlling the processes in the Fluid Body; we again in Phase Three discussed the importance of realizing that the tidal forces of the Health were inside the lesion field from the moment the trauma occurred.

In Phase Four we studied the Health again. This time we saw that it could "center us." The revelation is hard to assimilate, especially if you are intuitive. In order for us to see the Health, two elementals must occur. First, we must have a neutral mind. Second, the Health must enter that neutral and transmute our awareness into something connected to the Health and not our self-centeredness and its plan. Here we begin by the grace of the Health to experience a stillness that converts our senses. This stillness of the Tide (level three) is very different in its potency from the stillness that we saw previously. This is a Dynamic Stillness that is beyond rates and time. It is the edge of holy ground.

As we continued along in the Phases, we began to wait more easily for the Tide to center us, and as we became more neutral, the deeper Tide carried us into the House Under the Sea. We have seen many wonders along the way. Now in Phase Seven we come to the clear vision of several indwelling aspects of the Health. Love ... liquid light ... and a diamond matrix … the landscape is vast … and the principles of healing are even more substantial that what we have previously experienced.

A STILL SMALL VOICE

Rollin Becker, D.O., referred to these words many times. He insisted upon not adding to what the Tide transmitted. He asked us to "be still and know that I am God" (Psalm 46).

Dr. Becker was transmitting deep truths from the ancient wisdom of prophets. Psalm 46 is from King David when he is struck mute by the hand of God. God speaks to him and stills him. It is important to know that the "being still" in this case is not an act of human will. It is a highly elevated state of recognition of an individual by God, bringing that person into union and enlightenment. It is the most sacred state of being in all traditions.

At around 800 BC, Elijah, a poor desert dweller, enters the flock of the Judeo-Christian tradition. He obviously was impoverished by choice, like the desert dwellers who followed him years later. He was dressed for survival. He was not a priest. He was homeless, poor, and unkempt.

The belief of the Jews at that time was that God would speak only to the religious leaders. There was a firm hierarchy that one had to recognize in order to be in the presence of God. There was a belief in the "chosen few." Elijah confronted these inequalities.

He told the masses that God was within them, that God spoke as a still small voice in the heart of everyone. In his time, this was something new for most people, something that was contrary to thousands of years of tradition. Elijah awakens us to an indwelling place in God's house ... and a direct communication therein ... *what we call conscience*. The word "conscience" means to know together with God as one.

Why would Dr. Becker point us here to these ancient teachers? Is this not the Health we have pursued in our tradition?

There are no chosen few ... there is a voice ... a still and small voice ... how can we understand the wordless voice ... why is it so small, like an embryo? All these questions are answerable inside your own temple (the Health).

The greatest step is being centered by Deity ... letting yourself be healed, reconstructed by love.

God is love.

THE VOID, THE DYNAMIC STILLNESS, AND THE HEALTH

There are often questions about the above words. There are several meanings from different sources for each word depending on the context in which it is used.

In Biodynamics, the meaning of these words is in the context of their relationship within Primary Respiration as envisioned by W. G. Sutherland, D.O. The similarities between the Sutherland/Becker commentaries and the ancient teachings in all spiritual paths is impressive.

Meditation is a formatted activity, whereas contemplation is open-ended, without format except the yearning to experience the Divine. Sutherland's quest to find the fulcrum of Primary Respiration led him through a spiritual path that perhaps was not evident to him at first, but parallels the insights of many contemplatives, so I am comfortable speaking about these topics as a contemplative myself.

Sutherland's perceptual journey has been discussed in Phase One, but here we look at the milestones that one is taken to once the basics are mastered. The conversation with the Tide becomes more direct ... that is, one moves away from technique into the conscious dependency on the presence that animates what is called the Tide, the Mechanism, and Primary Respiration. This is what the work of Sutherland leads to for many of us who have "lived" the story.

My training, which began in 1966, included all the methods over forty years and led me to find the same teacher in my contemplative life as I did through Sutherland's work ... love animating creation with mercy and grace for all, a simple sentence that unveiled itself slowly as my eyes adjusted to the darkness (void) that was eventually illuminated by love. In the transparency that love imposes on us is a landscape that elevates the observer through its own death, and awakens an inversion of the senses to "see" the Health as it is animated and formed by the movement of eternity—the memory of which never fades even when a lesser darkness falls upon oneself. As we explore this landscape, these words will ring true, as they have through all of time.

Contemplation is risking fear and worldly success for the healing of oneself in hopes that the meaning of life will be better comprehended ... as the teacher comes, one sees that self-emptying love is at the center of everything and that self-fulfilling love can only start a small fire that becomes consumed by the fire that transmutes every second of existence into the fabric of eternity.

Our great teacher, Dr. Still, was not afraid of Divine love. The Science of Osteopathy is not limited to a belief in itself, but to the seeing of the laws of nature as they are, not as we construct them for profit or comfort. Those whom I have been closest to on this journey were strong enough to put the patient's well-being first and seek the most potent, noninvasive therapeutic tools available ... the Tide won first prize ... because it outperformed all other clinical trials (drugs, acupuncture, and homeopathy).

The void, the dynamic stillness, and the Health all have qualities that are unique and meaningful in clinical practice ... we will build a picture of these landscapes.

Beyond the inhalation and exhalation phases of the Tides, beyond the rates, lies a landscape that empties itself into all of life. The potency here exceeds the power of the potency we find at lower levels. It creates, destroys, animates, and heals in its passing. And yet it remains always the infrastructure of itself.

The story of these words begins with the dramatic movement from active to passive to neutral ... these words, although not commonly used, describe what people do when they treat.

The first step we teach in Biodynamics is the value of stillness as a fulcrum. This begins in Phase One and is seen as an end point for treatment.

In Phase Two we move to a different stillness, a stillness from which the breathing emerges and to which it returns. From this we find another stillness in Zone B (the fluid body) that unlocks the door to automatic shifting. This does not seem to confuse anyone. The profoundness of it seems normal and yet it is very profound ... an indwelling self-healing resource.

Soon we experience the Long-Tide. Here the stillness that crescendos during treatment fills Zone D. At first this is disarming as our senses are challenged. After several years, it all seems quite wonderful, but our sense of life is changing as we meet the natural senses that are not used much in the city or when one has one's own goals to accomplish. The natural senses are intelligent, creative, and innate.

To an aboriginal in the wilderness, the stillness that fills Zone D is the baseline of all function. The awareness of the horizon, Zone D, and the Long-Tide are in the perceptual foreground for the natural mind, not the background as they are for most educated people. The stillness has sacred movements as well as natural movements. The natural mind does not experience distance as we do; everything is near, and tapping in the heart is a phone line to the tribal circle. The little hearts of humans and the big heart that moves the stars all travel here. People grow in spirit in that world and come to a oneness that changes their role in the community. A hunter may eventually become a "monk," leaving his lodge and family to live alone, becoming a spiritual elder for his tribe. As one grows within this landscape of the Long-Tide, a deep sense of life emerges in the senses.

In order for us to move from the world of the Long-Tide closer to the cause, we must ask, "Where is the stillness that expresses the wholeness of Zone D? Where is the fulcrum?" Sometimes we do this because the landscape of the Long-Tide is not healing us as deeply as we feel is possible. We want to find the eternal and be whole.

When one looks for the fulcrum in Zone D, one does not know what is coming! If anything!

One leaves the instinct of nature for the spirit of the Health. The "my" is still in the equation. We step past the motions and geography of Zone D and we come to nothing! And I mean nothing.

There is no sensation at all. No stillness. It seems void like a corpse. There is no boundary, no sensation, nothing to trust or control or understand. The void is a place the ego avoids. This is the void. It can feel "dreadful," as Thomas Merton says in his books on contemplation.

Often, this absolute lack of anything causes fear. This comes from the ego losing its fulcrum. We expected to find something we can comprehend with ordinary knowledge. It is not what we imagined. Our sensory blindness blinds us.

Time passes and we begin to travel to the void over and over again. It is painful, opening the subconscious to weaknesses that lay hidden, exposing our selfishness and fears. We want to feel the Health, to feel Divine love, so we stay. What we meet is our smallness. We meet our own violence, which has been hidden by the cultural persona.

Some turn back, some stay and pray for help. It comes ... we realize that the void is a waiting place. A place where one does nothing but wait ... this becomes our first level neutral in a new world. Our sense of helplessness becomes rarefied into being still and not knowing. The void becomes a quiet place to retreat to for solitude. The battle that was ensuing ends in neutrality.

The vastness of the void becomes an ocean of presence and peace. We are embraced by a mantle of serenity that is boundless, kind, sheltering, sweet, tender, and loving.

The great mother has come to be with us as we become more whole in the healing presence of her love. We begin to heal in a way we could not imagine. A second neutral emerges. We are less active or passive. The reason for existing has changed. Just being in her presence is enough.

Something came to meet and heal us ... the void has become a meeting place ... then it becomes a resting place, a place of repose. The void becomes a dynamic stillness full of activity that heals us. It unveils the Health.

What appeared as a void becomes a place of pureness, inner poverty, and joy.

ZONE B AND THREE LEVELS OF STILLNESS

The ability to communicate and cooperate with the natural laws that frame the substance and activity of Zone B can lead to many wonderful clinical results.

Diagnostics in children often depend on seeing the relationships of Zone B to Zone A.

The normal Zone A (soma) is transparent to the Health and does not reflect anatomy any more than a muscle in neutral does. As you know, muscle in neutral feels like a bag of water.

Let's continue with this point of seeing Zone A and Zone B and their relationship. Can you draw the picture of Zone A and Zone B in this patient?

In the first chapter of *Philosophy of Osteopathy* by A. T. Still, D.O., he asks, What is anatomy? His reply needs your review, so you can see further than just the gross structure and understand our work in relation to the tradition Still began. Anatomy is a living wholeness of function and should be seen as a mystery of form, not static academic structure.

Additionally, my oldest Osteopathic friend, Eliott Blackman, once told me a story about wholeness, Zone B, and Osteopathy. The story is this: when in Kirksville in 1966 (Eliott's second year), he went to see Dr. Korr, our physiology teacher and author of *The Physiological Basis of Osteopathic Medicine*. He asked Dr. Korr, "Is the body a syncytium?" The answer came: "A visible segment is a segment in trouble."

A syncytiumis a group of cells acting as a single mass of protoplasm. In the fluid body there is no anatomy, no somatic segments, just protoplasm. When Zone B lesions, it becomes visible as Zone A. Zone

A transmutes under the influence of the Tide into Zone B.

As you evaluate your patient today, there will be a Zone A and a Zone B, but can you feel B without A? This skill is necessary.

As you find Zone B, can you feel its wholeness? It functions as one drop. There is no distance within its mind. As you sit where you are, everything is in your hands (literally).

Once the above is clear, we are going to explore the different levels of stillness and the landscapes in between.

The first level of stillness is the balance point between atmospheric pressure and the fluids in the body. We find this by sensing the air in the room and the same tone in the patient. There is no point of interface; it is a continuum. The stillness is a place of balance. It is calm. It is not a true stillness because it does not have any therapeutic potency.

Before we come to second level stillness, we pass through the space of the body chemistry, where we can read molecular disturbances. See what comes to you as you pass from the first level stillness into the breathing of the fluid body at two cycles per minute. It may feel odd. If you work at this, you can read a variety of chemical states.

Second level stillness is the fulcrum for the breathing, both primary and secondary. Let's begin by asking the question, "Does the fluid body in this patient respond to thoracic respiration?" In children and saints, the fluid body is suffused and powered by thoracic and Primary Respiration as one transmutative force. After checking thoracic respiration, then check for Primary Respiration and its influence on the fluid body. Next, see if the two respirations are relating to each other or if they are strangers.

Now we move to level two stillness. We sense the stillness from which and to which the breathing comes and goes. As we wait, the stillness moves into the foreground. Zone D comes into our awareness, automatically.

At this level we find the Long-Tide, an ocean breathing (Zone D). Sense the ocean without any Zone A, the house under the sea with all the doors and windows open.

We studied the next level of stillness in Phase Four, the dynamic stillness or third level stillness. This is also "the meeting place."

To witness this, one must go to the fulcrum for the Long-Tide.

As we come to the effort, we enter a void. In the context in which we are using it, the void is a place where we can perceive nothing but our own limits ... it is not pleasant. But if we have worked on this, the void is no longer a void, a place of tension as the ego dissolves, but a peaceful room in the House Under the Sea ... a waiting place where the Tide ripens our consciousness.

As our senses are converted by the presence in the house ... we begin to see the Health ... the beauty and transparency that we see in children.

Through this transparency comes a "wind" ... Divine and holy ... As we are touched by this stillness, we become aware of our own healing ... it has many dimensions, but it "holds us so completely" that we are renewed, purified, and able to move with the companionship of the host of the house ... the teacher has come ... as this awareness enters us, the whole world is seen as Health.

The movement of creation and eternity fills our abandoning vessel as a fourth level of stillness of angelic proportions and heralds the beginning of the return of the senses to the original state as an expression of the Health.

MEDITATION: FINDING THE HEALTH

Meditation is practicing truth. It involves active choices with the heart. In Phase One, we studied a kind of Yoga.

Yoga means "union with God."

Soma is an ancient word from Sanskrit … it relates to the idea of perfect form. It is not Zone A as we have studied it at universities.

Sensing your posture without changing it and sensing the soma is a very useful way to spend time with your Health.

Sense your posture as it is without changing it … then sense the perfected form … not with your imagination, but sense for the Health as it is in itself, near you.

Doing this for several minutes is restful and healing for Zone A and its dilemmas.

When Zone A senses this perfect form, it remembers the real soma, its connection with the Health and the Divine.

This blending of Zone A with the Health leads to physical changes in fluency that you can feel over several weeks.

Spend time with the Health. Become familiar with it and it will heal you in many ways.

Usually when we sense for the soma we feel a shadowy form of liquid light.

The soma can be beside Zone A, behind it, or in it—anywhere nearby.

Zone A has moved away from the soma … it is lost and imprisoned by the part of the soul that is worldly and self-centered.

The return to one's real self is healing for the many anxieties and emptiness that come when one is separate from the Health (soma).

All religions recognize the feeling of being broken away from the source of creation. With this insight from a Yogi, I began to see the soma form easily.

As I added this to my contemplation, it grew in meaning.

DR. A. T. STILL'S PHILOSOPHY OF IMMORTALITY

Dr. Andrew Taylor Still, the founder of the science of Osteopathy, gave a speech before the Missouri State and Mississippi Valley Osteopathic Association at Kirksville, Missouri, May 24, 1912. Here is a quote from it.

> Today I have no more fear of death than life. ... it will be a higher step ... necessary to man's spiritual perfection.
>
> When a chicken comes out of the shell ... he proves the perfection of the knowledge that is in him ...
>
> ... when I came to man he was both a physical and a mental dependent. He comes into the world a mental blank, and when he dies, he knows but little more, notwithstanding the days and years that he has spent in theological and scientific schools.
>
> I learned more from an old hen than all the theologians have ever taught me ... that our lives are in a body ... developing the spiritual man to make the step from mortality to immortality.
>
> Every evidence that I have found in all nature is that the God of life is an architect, a builder, an engineer ... and there is no perfection short of completion for which I think the spiritual man is retained in the physical body until nature says it is finished ...
>
> I will close by saying, "Know thyself and be at peace with God."

Andrew T. Still, “Philosophy of Immortality,” speech given at the Missouri State and Mississippi Valley Osteopathic Association at Kirksville, Missouri, May 24, 1912.

THE DYING PATIENT

Death is not extinguishing the light;
it is only putting out the lamp
because the dawn has come.
–Rabindranath Tagore

We all die. Some in the arms of love, some in despair. Often, we are present with patients during this phase of life and can support them through it as they transpire (breathe across).

As we enter the process of death, Primary Respiration changes. Its intention is to make the transition as easy as possible. One's consciousness is merging with the Health of the whole. The direction of ease during the time up to death is not visible to the Osteopathic hands unless they are sensing the Health.

In the turmoil of dying, the tissue quits. In metastatic disease, it can feel like "rotting" tissue.

As the metabolic systems fail and the patient wastes away, and the Long-Tide is swirling around the soma, the patient's pain is often unbearable and prolonged.

House calls are necessary.

One needs to feel if the Health or the suffering of the patient is augmented.

For example, a patient riddled with metastases cannot move without severe pain and despair.

Our hands must hold a flower, not a disease. This is not hard. Your training in Biodynamics will serve you well.

Patients that have a spiritual life (either formal or informal) have felt the Health. They often feel God's love and see death as the coming of eternal love and fire. This ignition, at death, in the old Christian teachings was called glorification. There may be other names.

Some patients are fearful. They believe they die, expire, succumb to lesions, and this makes for a different set of principles of treatment that we can discuss elsewhere.

This discussion is about patients who have felt a benevolent God's love and remember. A case history may help.

A wonderful, introverted elder woman was in love with the Great Mother of the Sea. She called her Mary. Her daily life was New Age in style, but her heart was open to Mary's love most of the time. She spoke only to me and her husband about this.

I knew her for fifteen years and watched her devotion begin and ripen. In the last several years before her cancer came, she was like a plant living next to a river ... she grew and grew ... until all she wanted was to feel the presence of Divine love and be with Mary.

She developed pancreatic cancer. It came quickly. In three months, the progress of the disease caused a crescendo of pain, everywhere. She was taking no medication, as the sense of Mary's love suffused her soma.

Her friends became a nuisance because they were afraid of death; this was straining her.

The disease was like a wildfire. One day she called me: "I cannot feel the love, the pain has overshadowed me. Can you come?"

Her reason for treatment was to feel the Health, the radiance of love ... she had many treatments and was often feeling a presence in the dynamic stillness at the end points.

When I saw her, she was exhausted, withdrawn, and crippled with pain. We had a treatment, and in twenty-four hours she called. "I can feel the love, there is no pain." She took no medication.

In the last months, I treated her five times. Each time, she easily found peace, talked with friends and helped them see her truth.

Several days after one treatment, I felt I should call her ... her husband said, "She is in bed all the time. She speaks to no one, but she said if you called she wanted me to hold the phone to her ear." ... He did ... She said, "I love you." In tears, I replied in kind. The last words between us were almost soundless and carried a solid caress that time cannot erase from our memory ... she died that day ... in the arms of her beloved Mary.

Our practical contains the principles that were used to help her and many others find a way to slip easily into the arms of the beloved. These principles are the same ones we have used with the dynamic stillness when we have slipped behind our breathing into the meeting place and waited. Now we move on toward feeling the Health and waiting.

THE TERMINALLY ILL PATIENT

House calls are necessary, especially near the end.

The patient should be comfortably positioned.

Any position of comfort is fine; the smallest pressure can cause pain.

Our hands must be embryonic, small and innocent.

There are several hints which may help you:

Tell your hands to remember the sensation of being touched by the Health ... use their memory!

Place your hands on gently with minimal surface contact, not off the body.

Feel your hands as they are and slowly decrease the voltage in stages until you feel the Health.

Your hands may surprise you as they become full of love—not yours, but from the Health.

If necessary, ask for the other pair of hands.

This step of sensing the Health in the patient is the most important, so explore what helps you perceive it.

Eventually your hands will remember the sensations of the Health with affection and clarity. There is a great ocean of help always nearby.

The patient is suffering intensely. Be neutral and work. Do not get attached to the suffering.

Because of the pain and mental despair, the patient's mind is shattered.

We need to bring them on center, to focus on one thing that will help organize a doorway to the meeting place (emptiness). From there, the breath of the Health will shift their consciousness. This is difficult for the patient ... it will take clear instruction and patience.

Ask the patient, "Can you see your breathing?" ... Usually, the response is "No" ... because the awareness is broken by the pain.

Tell them:

Try to see just a little of the breathing for a second. Do not fight the pain or distractions. Just find a little of the breathing.

Wait ... (do not stop sensing the Health, no matter what).

Wait more ... until Zone B changes ... a little.

Matching your voice to the Health, ask them ... can you feel your breathing?

They will say no.

Repeat to them, "Try to find your breathing. Do not fight. Just shift your mind to it. Slip in behind the pain and fear; go easy. Find the inhalation and the exhalation of the breathing.

Wait ... watch Zone B and stay with the Health.

After several conversations ... Zone B will crescendo, like an EV4. This means they have divided their attention and found the breathing. But when you inquire, they will still have pain ... Now we have *the pain and the breathing in the patient's awareness.*

Ask, "Can you see or feel an emptiness behind the breathing?" If no, then say, "Can you see a quietness behind your observer?" ... then you will get a yes ... all the answers are frail and painful.

Say, "Try to notice the breathing and the emptiness. Do not push the pain away. Just see the emptiness and the breathing at the same time."

Do not encourage them to connect the emptiness and the breathing.

Wait ... later Zone B and the Health will merge and transmute.

Wait.

Say, "How are you?" ... "Fine."

"Are you in pain?" ... "No."

Sweetly remove your contact, as the Health guides you ...

Call them the next day.

Notes

Dividing the attention between the breathing and the emptiness positions the observer to be transmuted by the Health.

Trying to go to the Health directly will not help but will only frustrate the patient and you.

Pain and fear are both emotions which transmute under the touch of the Health.

When the soma feels eternity one dies spiritually, and the pain and fear end as the body connects to the Health and the psyche begins to perish.

Visitors can be disruptive to the patient. Make sure they have only the company that they want.

AT THE CENTER OF OUR BEING

In *Conjectures of a Guilty Bystander* (1966), Thomas Merton writes:

> At the center of our being is a point of nothingness which is untouched by sin and by illusion, a point of pure truth, a point or spark which belongs entirely to God, which is never at our disposal, from which God disposes of our lives, which is inaccessible to the fantasies of our own mind or the brutalities of our own will. This little point of nothingness and of absolute poverty is the pure glory of God in us. It is so to speak his name written in us, as our poverty, as our indigence, as our dependence, as our sonship. It is like a pure diamond, blazing with the invisible light of heaven. It is in everybody, and if we could see it we would see these billions of points of light coming together in the face and blaze of a sun that would make all the darkness and cruelty of life vanish completely . . . I have no program for this seeing. It is only given. But the gate of heaven is everywhere.

QUOTES

I love my patients. I see God in their faces and their form.
A. T. Still, M.D., D.O.

When all the fulcrums are synchronized there will be peace and harmony.
W. G. Sutherland, D.O.

Seek the Health; anyone can find disease.
A. T. Still, M.D., D.O.

Health is the Imago Dei, breathed out by the Divine.
Hebrew scriptures

Wholeness is the smallest division of life.
Unknown

The Health does not end at death. The body is the second placenta. (paraphrased)
A. T. Still, M.D., D.O.

The perfect neutral is of the Health. Here, there is no perceptual tension. There is oneness with the Breath of Life and its wisdom.
James Jealous

THE HEALTH

Practical

This practical is exploratory and therapeutic.

Sense the whole of the suffering of the patient. This wholeness is the fabric of all the suffering. It is the sum total of the suffering without layers, places, or times. It feels like a black sheet or carpet.

It is not the person's sense of their suffering or the symptoms. It is a collective wholeness of separation.

Next, find the Health, another layer, a sweet, warm, honey-like substance. Sometimes we see only a piece of it. That is enough.

Notice the gap between the two.

Notice that the Health reaches into the suffering and not the other way around.

Let go of the Health on the inside of the patient.

Find the outside Health and its presence in the sea around us. What is it doing in relation to the suffering?

Now, add back the inner so we have both aspects of the Health (the outer and the inner) and the whole of the suffering.

What is the treatment like?

The Health is love, the most potent healing force of all. Lesions are transparent to it.

The outside presence is love eternal.

The inside is love eternal incarnate.

The suffering is temporal.

The gap is the lost memory.

The hand reaching over is the intercession of the Health into the suffering.

Eternal love incarnates.
Suffering comes, love increases.
Wholeness is sustained.

THE PATIENT'S SUFFERING AS A WHOLENESS

We have explored several avenues to a relationship with the Health.

This juxtaposition between the Health and the deformity is always present in us.

We have often spoken of the Health in the lesion, another Osteopathic truth.

Now we will sense the patient's suffering as a wholeness; we will simultaneously be aware of the Health and its wholeness. Following this, we will appreciate the gap that separates the suffering and the Health. As we view these aspects, we will also notice the hand of the Health reaching across the gap into the suffering (this is the therapeutic force in the Health moving into the lesion field).

After we see the above, we let go of this internal aspect of the Health and become aware of the outside presence of Primary Respiration. We will appreciate the whole of the suffering and the whole of the sea of love around us ... once we are aware of these two aspects, we will add back the wholeness of the internal Health. The suffering is sandwiched between the outer and inner aspects of the Health.

We have also looked at the perceptual arenas that we transit in our inner journey: the perfect neutral, empty of self, senses the void, where a shadow of another presence is developing into a real person, the Health, a place of eternal love. We studied how to guide a person into a place of meeting that love. Hopefully, we see that we are met in the void and touched by the Health; this Health carries us into the seeing of the new landscape. We meet the sweetness of unconditional love incarnate in us, as us. This begins a relationship. A friendship. This is the edge of oneness.

As we change, our breathing shifts. The separation of primary and thoracic respiration narrows and the reunion is imminent. Our meditation will embrace the breathing of thoracic respiration, the void, and the breathing of the sea of love. The two breaths may touch, merge, and pour into each other. Usually, the primary breathing suffuses the thoracic, but not the other way around. Here, much changes as we enter into self-emptying as opposed to self-fulfilling beingness.

We become aware of memory eternal.

BREATHING

As you know, rates express breathing.

The breathing changes as we move deeper within the activities of Primary Respiration. As the rate slows, the breathing becomes more subtle ... rich ... and ... potent ... at times stopping.

This is also true of thoracic respiration, which changes its pattern as we come to rest in neutrals at different levels.

Thoracic respiration has many nonmechanical qualities, which we will continue to explore here and in Phase Eight.

We can watch thoracic respiration and its landscapes. This will lead us into places of great meaning and serenity.

We begin by being aware of the inhalation and exhalation as the flow of life without a sense of ownership, i.e., "my breathing."

This movement of life is not ours ... it is given to us for existence.

As we watch it move, we can also watch our own tensions change as the ease of respiration increases. The pauses that appear are also doorways to something deeper, hidden behind a veil.

When we settle into the awareness of breathing, we can ask, "Where is the fulcrum?" as Sutherland so often did in his classes ... where is this breathing coming from ... who is breathing ... where is cause ... and wait ... we can sense a quiet room from which the movements of breathing come and go ...

As we concentrate on this quiet room ... it moves into the foreground and the breathing moves into the background ...

We find ourselves in a room ... in a house ... under the sea.

When we first came here it was a void, dark and scary. But now we know, it is as the foyer in a house under the sea, where one can wait for the owner of the house who will come to greet us.

As we wait, we rest ... pausing ... breathlessness occurs for brief periods. The house is great, and in it we can hear the Master asleep, breathing.

The master's breath comes to us and centers our breathing in the Health ... as one breath ... centered ... moving up the center, not in (out).

Some have called this the embryonic breath.

BREATHING SYNCHRONIZATION

As we wait with the breath, time passes. The breathing becomes simple; the sound changes; there are pauses, moments of breathlessness that are pure and effortless. These pauses are points of meeting the Health. We are being synchronized by an indwelling healing presence.

Breathing like a sleeping infant.

Neutral in the house.

Zone A becomes transparent.

The house is under the sea, and the sea breathes through it. We come to Primary Respiration. Breathing that has no boundary, coming through everything without touching it or diminishing itself.

We become aware of the house, and two breaths.

Waiting, we are resting the little mind.

Are the two breaths suffusing each other in both directions?

THE HEALTH IN ONESELF

We have many different selves, some positive, some negative, and they all want us to follow them. They want our attention.

The Health in us is very near, and waiting for neutral to actively engage in healing us.

We are unaware of most of this, so we might believe that we are not in contact with the Health even when we are.

We may think, "Yesterday I felt the Health but today I cannot." This is not true. The Health is always there.

When in doubt, look inside yourself.

Can you feel a sweet, warm, honey-like substance?

Is it isolated from Zone A or is it interfacing with A and treating? What is it doing?

Sometimes we find the Health where we least expect to.

It is possible to feel the Health even when you can't feel it, because there are two observers, not one.

One that knows and one that does not want to know ... both are always accessible ... if you believe you cannot feel it, you will not ... take a moment to look behind your sense of "not feeling it" ... look behind the veil of your belief ... what's in the background?

SUNRISE

There are many landscapes within the dynamics of Primary Respiration. As we become aware of the transparency of the whole, all landscapes will become more visible. Now, let's begin with the darkness and stillness of the "Ocean of the Dynamic Stillness."

NEUTRAL OF THE HEALTH

Formlessness

Practical

Sense the fluid body as a whole, One Transparent Drop Breathing

Wait

Sense the Long-Tide, inside and outside.

Wait

Sense the Dynamic Stillness inside and outside as a rich dark substance, like onyx.

Wait

Wait for the dawn.

Sense the patient as a whole.

Sense the embryonic plate of liquid light.

Wait.

What transpires?

Formlessness is a place of metamorphosis.

The Perfect Zone B

Liquid light

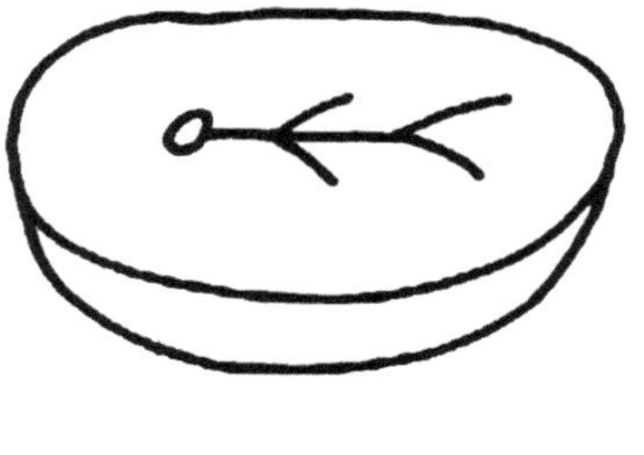

THE NEUTRAL OF THE HEALTH

To our concrete minds, many of the activities of Primary Respiration make no sense. Yet they are everyday occurrences in nature.

Transmutation

Transmutation can be seen as the change of one kind of species into another.

The drama of this change as it occurs is unsettling for our compensations, because one develops a sense of security around one's losses. We try to build a "safe" life and security in the socioeconomic face of any given culture. The cultural patterns are predictable … the Tide is not predictable … sometimes there are transmutations that seem impossible.

Outside your cultural world is activity that only mystics and children notice. The white spot on a milkweed leaf grows into a caterpillar; that seems quite remarkable in itself. Later, the caterpillar attaches to another leaf and spins a cocoon. Soon it becomes a green slime. It has become a Zone B. The cocoon is transparent. You can see a shadowy figure emerging from the green slime. It grows into a new form and gets bigger. The cocoon opens. A monarch butterfly emerges to dry in the sun. It must wait before it flies. Waiting is a pause. Then it flies. It travels three to six thousand miles in the turbulence of a hurricane season to a tree where its parents came from in South America. How many changes are required to bring us home to our origin? Try to let change be easy; it has direction.

Formlessness is a neutral.

We have seen that the Perfect Zone B (Health) somehow dissolves the patient. It seems impossible, but for a second the patient has become neutral in the most complete manner.

This transmutation is as important to our unfolding as it is to the unfolding of the monarch butterfly. The drama of healing, of being in and through neutral, is happening before your very eyes. After Zone B encapsulates around the patient, there is a secret meeting. As the treatment ends, the patient reforms. All this is visible.

There are many mystical commentaries on metamorphosis (see Ovid). The metaphors linger as a resource of change.

Think how different the world is for a caterpillar, a butterfly, and an egg.

Our consciousness will change in ways that will be very different from the transformations that come from personal effort and psychological reorientation. Metamorphosis is a transmutation, the power of which does not come from us.

Transmutation occurs naturally in the natural world ... it occurs in us ... medical science shows no awareness of this ... however, Sutherland clearly reports it.

The neutral of the Health is empty of form or will. If perchance we fall into it, we will feel a sweet, soft transparency ... a room ... outside "in the streets" is human nature and its projections (yours and others) ... in this cocoon we find a mysterious joy, even when we are insulted by others or by our own lower self ... a joy ... not a loud joy ... a soft one.

We change.

It's the not-yet in the now,

the taste of the fruit that does not-yet exist,

hanging the blossom on the bough.

Laurens van der Post, Venture to the Interior

Eternity is a child playing ...

–Heraclitus

THE MATRIX OF THE HEALTH

The word matrix is used here to denote an internal latticework within the substance of the Health. We hear about this from Sutherland in his many references to the unerring precision of the Tide. We also know from Blechschmidt and other embryologists that the growth process lays out the perfect matrix as an infrastructure upon which life unfolds. This latticework is like a skeletal system for the blueprint of life. The geometry is perfect and full of intersecting lines and points of intersection we call fulcrums.

The matrix appears as golden lines. We witnessed some of this in Phase Four when we worked with the pregnant pelvis.

When we lesion, our functions move off these perfect lines and begin to function on "false lines" or false midlines. These lines are black. They are set up by the Health to protect the whole from destruction by the stress that overwhelmed the organism.

I recommend you read: *The Power of Limits: Proportional Harmonies in Nature, Art, and Architecture*, by Gyorgy Doczi (1981), about the mathematical development of the matrix.

THE MATRIX

Practical

We will work with the brain.

- There are two matrices, one Healthy, the other a lesion field. The Health is golden lines, and the lesion is black lines.
- The patient must first express neutral. Wait until they do before proceeding with diagnostics.
- Find the golden line(s) and the black line(s). One line is enough because both the Health and the lesion are wholes.
- Divide your attention between the two contrasting lines.
- Wait until you feel (and see) a communication between them.
- Do not encourage a connection. Do not encourage movement.
- Why not? Because there is already a connection. When you as a person feel your Health, what happens? Most people feel a need to return, as does the lesion ... this, then, is the return and the treatment that is self-regulating ... we only reconnect the memory in the lesion.
- Call the patient in three days.

Perfect Brain, on Matrix

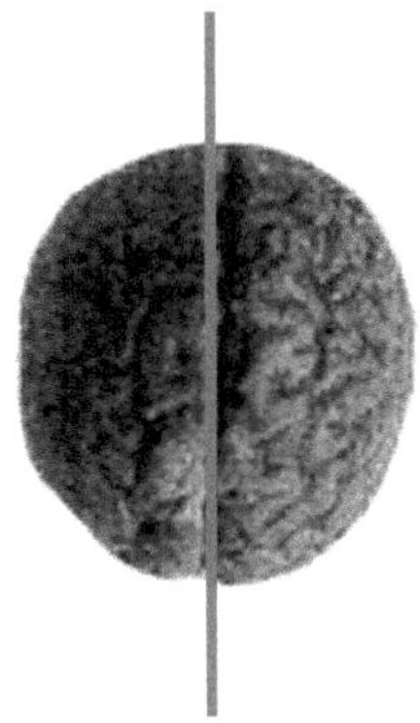

Lesioned Brained with False Midline (Compensatory)

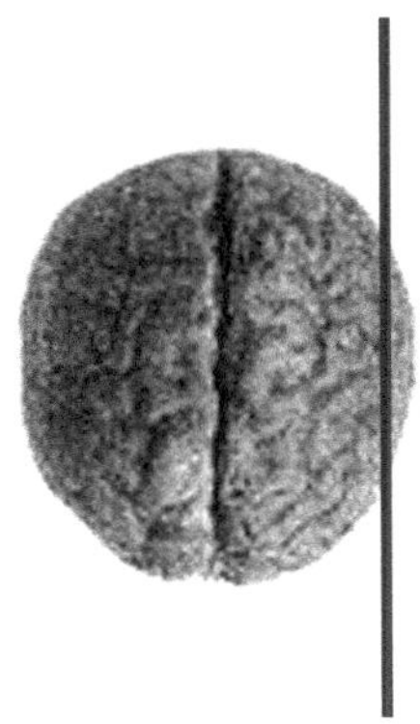

Both Lines and Lesioned Brain

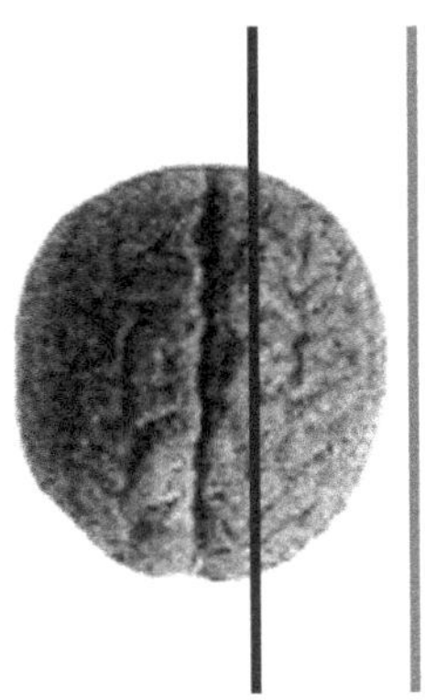

A CASE HISTORY

A patient was seen at the request of a family member. The time was short, and I had to fit her into the day. She was visiting from out of town.

She had had brain surgery near the sensory-motor strip eleven years before. The surgery saved her great suffering but left her with limitations: left facial and left upper extremity numbness, loss of motor function of the left hand, loss of muscle strength in the left upper extremity…

The patient was already in neutral when I placed my hands on her. I commented on this. She was a woman of faith.

The treatment was exactly as I described for the practical, nothing more. The duration of the whole visit was fifteen minutes, including introductions.

She left and returned to another part of the country. She wrote me several weeks later:

"I am sure this will not be news to you, but I am experiencing more feeling in my left hand, and I am back to some of my exercises I learned eleven years ago to strengthen my muscles. This was something that was totally out of the realm of possibility for me, and words cannot express my gratitude. I can now close my left eye without closing my right eye. That is pretty amazing to me. I can also pick up paperclips pretty quickly as opposed to straining and struggling with my left hand."

The Tide is a mystery that we can become comfortable with … but it is not predictable or understandable. The principles of Osteopathy work.

LOVE IS SPEECHLESS

We find many principles along this Osteopathic path.

We make effort to grow, and we do. It is self-fulfilling love that carries us.

When we follow that love we go a long way and become "filled."

Then we enter the house under the sea, where our love for life is not enough.

The master comes and empties us of this "fullness."

Then we are empty of any knowing that got us here, to this special place.

Then the teacher, who is the master, touches you.

Love is poured into you that only the little you can tolerate.

But the taste is different. It is self-emptying love.

Love from the Health empties itself to help us travel the rest of the way.

The heart meets the "heart that sees only one Health everywhere."

Then love flows through us.

We may not feel it because the peace it gives us is so severe. This state is satiety. When the contrast is gone, the feeling of love for anything is gone. It is unconditional. We receive as much as what flows ... all we notice is an inner peace and oneness.

COMMENTS

Beyond rates is soundless breathing.

In rapture, we are carried from one place to another.

In ecstasy we are unaware of external surroundings.

Imagination is the genius of the creative faculty of the mind, and what may be its highest aspect.

Syncytium: many cells acting as a single mass of protoplasm

Transmutation can be seen as the altering of form from one species to another species; a complete conversion.

Universe: one word

Senseless: in the presence of beauty eternal, moronic behavior

Conscience: clean intuition, wisdom

Perception is malleable.

At death, the range of motion of the bones increases. Maybe because the ego dies.

Movement in nature empowers the attention to divide and deepen in all directions. Be distracted when you are touched by the Tide. Find beauty and the transparency will increase.

We need the free will to be neutral, not controlled will.

Rationalizations are life-threatening.

When we find our Health, we heal ourselves and our community.

We are guided by deeply humbled sincerity, not skill. We come to treasure powerlessness, innocence, and the presence of love.

Patience will reveal myriads of self-deception. This helps.

Emotions, feeling, and inspiration are all at different levels.

With love upon us, our enemies are loved. We see them as God's children.

All the Zones are inside the patient, as well as outside ... inside the patient are all the landscapes of Primary Respiration.

Choosing service in today's world requires a community for support.

When we find the Health we can be deceived easily, until it becomes as near as our breath. Discernment requires knowing what the intention of God's will is, not what is safe or what moves other people.

There are two fluid bodies: one in the Health and one that can lesion.

Love creates love, holy fire.

Wisdom is self-emptying love.

Feelings are self-fulfilling love that can give direction to finding the void where we are fulfilled, then emptied.

Emotions are unfulfilling, self-centered love.

Intellect is a little mind caught in time.

Intuition is an emotional understanding of the truth.

Instinct is the body hearing the Health.

We are one spiritual substance; feel this.

One substance, not liquid light and darkness, one.

Jeremiah chapter 1, verse 5.

Neutral in the Health is the place of dynamic interchange.

Psalm 46.

RECOMMENDED READING

Always reread Dr. Still and Dr. Sutherland.
Dr. Becker's books are excellent, especially now.

The Great Mystics Have a Lot to Teach Us about the Health and Coming to It:

Saint John of the Cross: his Collected Works are easily found; deep, long, intense

Saint Teresa of Avila: *The Interior Castle*; intense

Jean-Pierre de Caussade: *Abandonment to Divine Providence*; short but excellent

Martin Laird: *Into the Silent Land*, an excellent concise book on contemplation

Camille Helminski: *Rumi Daylight: A Daybook of Spiritual Guidance*

Jewish wisdom: *The Book of Wisdom* ... exceptional

Shaila Catherine: *Focused and Fearless: A Meditator's Guide to States of Deep Joy, Calm, and Clarity*

Ramana Maharshi: Anything he wrote

Stories That Open Doors:

Helen Luke: *Kaleidoscope*; lots of old stories

Laurens van der Post: *The Heart of the Hunter*

IGNITION

Each of us embraces a divine spark.

It keeps alive our yearning for perfection.

It shines light into our confusion.

It warms the embryo.

Its presence gives us patience.

It illuminates the darkness.

It reveals the way... home.

J.J. Fall 2001

In the noonday of mystery they gathered

By the side of a deep phantom well.

Wooing the fates that were hidden,

Listen, the future to tell.

Faintly the whisper was wafted

As incense upon the night dew:

Be brave, be courageous, be honest,

To your heart ever be true.

Andrew Taylor Still

A DEFINITION OF LOVE

Dr. A. T. Still, December 1896

Love is the true color of life
When moved by contact of eye,
Oceans of inexpressible acts of strife,
Come from friend, man or wife.

It has not yet been described by man,
It binds man to man, how? Unknown,
It comes, never to leave again,
It fills our minds to feast when alone.

It comes and stays,
A loving flame of soul,
And asks no change of ways,
But to find a friend and unfold.

It is the odor for smell, taste and sight,
Comes with self, as part of laws,
Comes gentle, and never with might;
Without a word of self or cause.

To embrace, to fondle, and draw to
Itself to feed the being unseen,
That law of life only can make or do,
Willing to allow nothing to stay between.

Love begins in self and ends in you,
And asks to roam no farther during life,
Is content when found in friend, child or wife;
And no other ending can even partly do.

Nov. 26, 1920

Dear Dr. Wentworth,

I am sure glad the board reached you in due time, and I do hope the man will give you a good gavel.

It gives me great pleasure in being able to give the Maine Osteopaths this small token of love and friendship in the name of my dear father Andrew Taylor Still.

His simple dignity, his upright life, his native pride, his impatience with shame, his clear and kindly heart all marked him for what he was. He truly loved his fellowman. The poor and distressed were nearest to his heart. He gladly turned aside from the great to help the humble. "He loved to love and be loved."

Sincerely,
Blanche Still Laughlin

This board was part of the baseboard from his own room.

LENGTH, WIDTH, BREADTH, AND DEPTH

One can become highly skilled and still not witness directly the tremendous power of the Breath of Life. One can develop a "feel for the dramatic subtleties of the fluid potencies" and even the spiritual fulcrum in the room, and yet the depth may not invade one's perception. Depth, an endless ocean of love.

Sensory skills can develop as a strictly biological phenomenon for the clinician and the teacher. We can cooperate and use the forces of life. We can feel as a "helper" but without sensing the depth of the Tide. One can work and never strike gold, the awestruck sense of the wide, mysteriously personal and universal embrace of an undying concern for the wellness of all: love. Not my love, but the love that the Tide, the Breath of Life, has for each creation.

Being aware of this love as a distinct quality of the Tide as it comes and keeps coming, even in one's darkest hour, is the greatest gift of this moment. The depth appears as the foundation of the entire process; one surrenders deeply and the treatment is out of one's hands. Less and less and less, only the infinitely small remains to be done.

A spark, a slight motion and the healing emerges, deeply; body, soul, spirit feel it as one. The psychological world ends, it dies into the depth. The questions stop, and both the clinician and the patient see into the truth. We are loved, deeply. Nothing more.

Much disease is supported by fear and separation. Our treatment, as W. G. Sutherland proposed, is from a great healing stillness. To Dr. Sutherland goes our gratitude for his uncompromising memory and direction—Amen.

WRITINGS BY JAMES JEALOUS, D.O.

I sit down to share these moments
With you. Which voice do I speak
With; the transient or the beloved.

Perhaps living in the natural world
Becomes the answer.

I have stories, new horizons and yet
The warming silence fills the moment
And stills my voice.

I am waiting to hear the long conversation
That unfolds when the sun rises
In the hearts of those who live in the sea.

Now is so greatly felt
My thoughts Yield into being.
The given.

One is never tempted to leave.
Not anymore. Winning is no
Reward if one poisons one's own home.

Drops of love, not enough for
Complete formlessness, but enough to
Know it shall be!

I am losing my desire.
A whisper forging steel
Even this little is forever.

To speak the transient is to be transient.
To speak of Him as he walks by
Is to live in speechlessness

James Jealous, D.O.
March 25, 2003

BIODYNAMICS OF OSTEOPATHY BOOK SERIES

This book is one of a series of twelve *Biodynamics of Osteopathy* books. It is recommended that you read the whole series in order, as each book builds on the understanding from prior books. It is also recommended that you seek experienced teachers and mentors to help you experience the full depth of the information given.

The full series is as follows:

Phase One is about involuntary motion, which is motion present in the whole and in the lesion. We learn to synchronize with the breathing of Primary Respiration before we approach any treatment. This synchronization is the key to working with stable rates and not irritating the system. The principle of synchronizing with a healthy aspect of the patient suffuses the whole teaching program. This synchronization shifts our awareness to a different level of receptivity, which allows us to see Primary Respiration rather than the lesion field, and this eventually leads us to an understanding of the intention of Primary Respiration.

Phase Two is about communication with the natural laws of healing that surround activity at 2 to 3 cycles per minute. We synchronize with the breathing of Primary Respiration and also add the skill of sensing the fulcrum, the Stillness through which the breathing creates form and function. It is a different kind of synchronization from that in Phase One, shifting our awareness more deeply. As this occurs, the treatment automatically expresses itself. The end point of treatment, when compared with Phase One, reveals several differences. We find this kind of synchronization works exclusively with the fluid body and the outcome of treatment is more complete than when working with tissue alone.

Phase Three is centered around the activities of the Long Tide (100 second cycle). We explore an indwelling therapeutic force already present in the lesion field. We learn that the dural system is not made-up of three sickles but rather a series of folds in a sac, arising during growth and development. We see the relationship between the upper and lower dural sacs, awakening us to the independence of two separate tentorium cerebelli. We discover that zone D, the horizon, and the Wire (along which the Long Tide moves during its intended therapeutic course) are all linked as natural laws pertaining to this level of Primary Respiration.

Phase Four focuses on the Midline, a place where the spatial relationships are expressed as a whole. It synchronizes and centers us in such a way that we become aware of Zone D and the Dynamic Stillness. The Third Level Stillness in Phase Four is different from the Stillness in the other Phases – we are centered by the Stillness at the center of creation. Our intention is replaced by the intention of the Tide which can facilitate our spiritual path.

Phase Five is about *the face*. As we approach the face, we use all of the principles that we have learned in Phase One, Two, Three, and Four. We work with automatic shifting and notice differences from how the face is viewed by older models within Osteopathy in the Cranial Field. As we synchronize with the therapeutic presence of the Long Tide we see what we can learn about the face from that landscape. We also work with Seams, Dynamic Stillness, and Ignition.

Phase Six is a continuation of our journey into the Wholeness that generates life and delivers therapeutic forces that transmute lesions once Neutral is expressed. It is a mixture of activities centered around the outside presence of Primary Respiration as something that is a non-biological force and that has a persona. We will also continue to explore seams and then move on to the extremities, first in the embryological terms and then as Sutherland taught them in his work called PowerPoints. Phase 6 is a time to build your understanding of the Tide and refine your skills.

Phase Seven highlights the Health. Dr. Still's famous comment "Find the Health; anyone can find disease," has plagued many minds over the last century. We come to the clear vision of several indwelling aspects of the Health: Love ... liquid light ... and a diamond matrix. A approach to the terminally ill and dying patient is addressed. In the somatic sensation of the Tide passing through the House Under the Sea, our awareness is transmuted by the Health. The lesion is seen as a precognitive act of the Health. Thoracic Respiration, Primary Respiration, and Ignition are as One. The landscape is vast ... and the principles of healing are even more substantial than we have previously experienced..

Phase Eight is a deeper exploration of seams, balanced rhythmic interchange, and the Flame of Intention as a therapeutic modality. Phase Eight is the culmination of our awareness of Wholeness, and ultimately brings us to the Divine Presence, Unconditional Love and Oneness. The living Tide dominates the awareness while forms move to the background. One feels the Breath of Creation in oneself as the Center of Wholeness. One feels the Unfoldment of oneself as one is Created. Our consciousness is a gift; we do not own it and if we try to control it we lose Wholeness.

Phase Nine is when we are able to fully evaluate and treat the Central Nervous System and the Eye. We also address Fire and the therapeutic modality of the Shakedown. True action is moved from Love and makes our perception exist. This Love is self-emptying and by its nature allows us to Serve as part of the Perfect. Perception can be used to Serve something other than ourselves. We have attempted to enter this balance point between the Perfect and the Disease ... it is a point where the whole of everything is suspended by Love as it works to incarnate the Complete. In the balance point of everything is The Intention of the Tide following the movement of the distortion back to a True relationship with the Blueprint of Life.

Pediatrics One explores how children grow as a whole, not in parts as we sometimes believe. Children live in the Direction of Ease of motion present in their fluid metabolic fields, otherwise they get uncomfortable and require assistance. Does your treatment directly support the whole, or does it assume to support the whole? We realize children are not adults and cannot be treated as adults are. We approach the therapeutic modality of the "Meeting Place", prenatal and postnatal periods, the treatment of the pelvis during pregnancy, fetal malposition and labor.

Pediatrics Two is where we deepen in the perceptive awareness necessary to approach the treatment of children. We deepen in our appreciation of Wholeness, the three levels of Stillness and the "Meeting Place". We approach "Desert Neutral", where therapeutics pass into the neutral substance, and a mystery unfolds as the breath of Divine love cascades as a therapeutic force across a night desert landscape, filling and leaving behind no visible effects. We further address treatment of the pelvis and the uterus during pregnancy. We explore thoracic and Primary Respiration in children, and the Family Circle.

Pediatrics Three is where we continue to study the therapeutic Flow of Attention. We deepen in Third Level Stillness and the Meeting Place. The Meeting Place is easily misinterpreted ... our observer must be so still and neutral that the process can be seen as it happens. The central nervous system in the child can be finally approached for evaluation and treatment. We explore teething and also the "locked up head". We use the therapeutic modality of the Flame of Intention, and its connection to the Breath of Life. Everything is transparent to the Breath of Life.

ABOUT THE AUTHOR

James Jealous, D.O. (1943–2021), was an osteopathic physician, teacher, and writer. His life's work was founding and developing **Biodynamics of Osteopathy**, a unique methodology he established within the field of osteopathy, following the lineage of Dr. A.T. Still and Dr. W.G. Sutherland.

He was born in Saco, Maine, and since his father was an osteopathic physician, he was around osteopathy from an early age. He studied at Kirksville College of Osteopathic Medicine in Missouri (now the A.T. Still University of Health Sciences), graduating in 1970. He then set up practice in rural Maine as an osteopathic primary care physician.

Over time, Dr. Jealous saw parallels between the work of embryologist Dr. Erich Blechschmidt and that of osteopathic physician Dr. William Garner Sutherland. This inspiration led him to create his own body of work. In the early 1990s, he began teaching "A Biodynamic View of Osteopathy in the Cranial Field," which, as he developed his specific methodology, was refined to "Biodynamics of Osteopathy."

A deeply spiritual person, he felt most at home in the natural world and was an avid fisherman and hiker.

For more information, please visit:
https://BiodynamicsOfOsteopathy.com

There is a wind passing through …
it is the motion of creation,
the eternal motion of Divine love.